THIS PLANNER

Belongs To:

I'm PREGNANT!

DUE DATE

HOW I FOUND OUT

MY REACTION

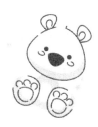

WHAT I AM MOST EXCITED ABOUT

WHO I TOLD FIRST

WHAT I WANT YOU TO KNOW

MY BIRTH PLAN *Ideas*

WHO I WANT IN THE DELIVERY ROOM:

TYPE OF BIRTH

☐ VAGINAL   ☐ WATER BIRTH

☐ C-SECTION   ☐ VBAC

THOUGHTS ABOUT BIRTH AND WHAT IS MOST IMPORTANT TO ME

GETTING READY FOR THE BIG DAY: TO DO

NOTES & IDEAS (lighting, music, etc.)

40 Weeks

PREGNANCY Tracker

Keep track of how you're feeling every week of your pregnancy.

APPOINTMENT *Tracker*

Keep track of your pre-natal classes and doctor appointments.

DATE	TIME	ADDRESS	PURPOSE

BABY SHOPPING *List*

Start planning for the arrival of your baby by using the shopping list below.

Undershirts

Socks

Pajamas

Sweaters

Onesies

Hats

Bibs

Blanket

Diaper Bag

Mitts

Diapers

Booties

Receiving Blankets

Crib Sheet

Wash Cloths

Towels

_____

_____

_____

Crib

Bassinet

Baby Bath tub

Car Seat

Stroller

High Chair

Play Pen

Baby Swing

Monitor

Change Table

Rocking Chair

Night Light

Mobile

Bouncer

Nail Clippers

Teething Toys

Baby Wipes

Diaper Pail

_____

_____

Bottles

Bottle Liners

Nursing Bra & Pads

Breast Pump

Formula

Pacifiers

Bottle Brush

Burp Cloths

Bottle Sanitizer

Nipples

Baby Powder

Baby Wipes

_____

_____

_____

_____

_____

_____

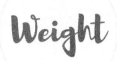

Weight PREGNANCY Tracker

♥♥♥ ♥♥♥ **Weight Tracker Chart** ♥♥♥ ♥♥♥

It's important to keep track of your weight throughout your pregnancy.
Record your weight in the chart below every week, starting at week 4.

WEEKLY WEIGHT TRACKER

4	12	20	28	36
5	13	21	29	37
6	14	22	30	38
7	15	23	31	39
8	16	24	32	40
9	17	25	33	
10	18	26	34	
11	19	27	35	

NOTE According to the American Pregnancy Association, pregnant women should consume up to 300 more calories a day. Further, healthy eating is critical to your baby's development which means you should make sure to maintain a well-balanced diet, high in nutrients and proteins.

HEALTHY FOOD Ideas

VEGETABLES & LOW SUGAR FRUIT	PROTEINS	COMPLEX CARBS	HEALTHY FATS	SUPPLEMENTS
Leafy greens (spinach, etc.)	Organic meat	Beets	Avocado	Vitamin D
Broccoli	Liver	Carrots	Olive Oil	Fish Oil
Cauliflower	Bone Broth	Sweet Potatoes	Coconut Oil	Algae Oil
Cabbage	Beans	Yams	Yogurt	Probiotics
Asparagus	Lentils	Parsnips	Almonds	Ginger Pills
Cucumber	Flax Seed	Turnips	Mixed Nuts	Licorice Root
Mushrooms	Pumpkin Seed	Pumpkin	Soybean	Magnesium
Celery	Chia Seed	Buckwheat	Olives	Krill Oil
Radish	Salmon	Brown Rice	Nut butter	Iron Pills
Grapefruit & Melon	Herring	Squash		
Berries (all kinds)				
Peaches (with skin)				

Tracker PRE-NATAL *Visits*

Important Dates

Keep track of your pre-natal appointments and include a summary of each visit.

DATE	SUMMARY OF APPOINTMENT
HOW FAR ALONG?	
YOUR WEIGHT	
BLOOD PRESSURE	
FETAL HEART RATE	
DOCTOR	
NOTES:	

NEXT APPOINTMENT.:

DATE	SUMMARY OF APPOINTMENT
HOW FAR ALONG?	
YOUR WEIGHT	
BLOOD PRESSURE	
FETAL HEART RATE	
DOCTOR	
NOTES:	

NEXT APPOINTMENT.:

DATE	SUMMARY OF APPOINTMENT
HOW FAR ALONG?	
YOUR WEIGHT	
BLOOD PRESSURE	
FETAL HEART RATE	
DOCTOR	
NOTES:	

NEXT APPOINTMENT.:

1-13 Weeks

FIRST *Trimester*

Journal your thoughts and feelings during each trimester so you can later reflect on your pregnancy journey.

HOW I FELT DURING MY FIRST TRIMESTER

MY FAVORITE MEMORIES

SYMPTOMS & CRAVINGS

ENERGY

♡ ♡ ♡ ♡ ♡ ♡

SLEEP

♡ ♡ ♡ ♡ ♡ ♡

CRAVINGS

♡ ♡ ♡ ♡ ♡ ♡

MOODS

♡ ♡ ♡ ♡ ♡ ♡

TO DO LIST: 1st TRIMESTER

FIRST TRIMESTER *Photos*

MEMORIES ARE FOREVER

14-27 Weeks

SECOND Trimester

HOW I FELT DURING MY SECOND TRIMESTER

ENERGY

SLEEP

CRAVINGS

MOODS

MY FAVORITE MEMORIES

TO DO LIST: 2nd TRIMESTER

SYMPTOMS & CRAVINGS

SECOND TRIMESTER *Photos*

MEMORIES ARE FOREVER

28-40 Weeks

THIRD Trimester

HOW I FELT DURING MY THIRD TRIMESTER

ENERGY

SLEEP

CRAVINGS

MOODS

MY FAVORITE MEMORIES

TO DO LIST: 3rd TRIMESTER

SYMPTOMS & CRAVINGS

THIRD TRIMESTER *Photos*

MEMORIES ARE FOREVER

MY BABY *Shower*

BABY SHOWER PHOTOS

GAMES PLAYED

ON THE MENU

HIGHLIGHTS & MEMORIES

MY BABY *Shower Gifts*

Keep track of your baby shower gifts and send thank you notes

NAME	GIFT	ADDRESS	SENT?

NURSERY *Planner*

COLOR SCHEME IDEAS:

ITEM TO PURCHASE	PRICE	NOTES

FURNITURE IDEAS

DECORATIVE IDEAS

BABY NAME *Ideas*

TOP 3 BOY NAMES

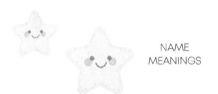

NAME
MEANINGS

TOP 3 GIRL NAMES

NAME
MEANINGS

BABY NAME RESOURCES (LIST YOUR FAVORITE PARENTING & PREGNANCY WEBSITES):

OTHER BOY NAME POSSIBILITIES	OTHER GIRL NAME POSSIBILITES

HOSPITAL Checklist

FOR ME	FOR PARTNER	FOR BABY

PREGNANCY SHOPPING *List*

BABY CLOTHING	SUPPLIES/MEDICATION	FURNITURE/TOYS

FIRST TRIMESTER SHOPPING	SECOND TRIMESTER SHOPPING	THIRD TRIMESTER SHOPPING

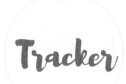

Tracker FETAL *Movement*

Starting around week 16, keep track of when you feel your baby move.

WEEK 16	TIME	NOTES
MON		
TUE		
WED		
THU		
FRI		
SAT		
SUN		

WEEK 17	TIME	NOTES
MON		
TUE		
WED		
THU		
FRI		
SAT		
SUN		

WEEK 18	TIME	NOTES
MON		
TUE		
WED		
THU		
FRI		
SAT		
SUN		

WEEK 19	TIME	NOTES
MON		
TUE		
WED		
THU		
FRI		
SAT		
SUN		

WEEK 20	TIME	NOTES
MON		
TUE		
WED		
THU		
FRI		
SAT		
SUN		

WEEK 21	TIME	NOTES
MON		
TUE		
WED		
THU		
FRI		
SAT		
SUN		

WEEK 22	TIME	NOTES
MON		
TUE		
WED		
THU		
FRI		
SAT		
SUN		

WEEK 23	TIME	NOTES
MON		
TUE		
WED		
THU		
FRI		
SAT		
SUN		

WEEK 24	TIME	NOTES
MON		
TUE		
WED		
THU		
FRI		
SAT		
SUN		

Tracker FETAL Movement

WEEK 25	TIME	NOTES
MON		
TUE		
WED		
THU		
FRI		
SAT		
SUN		

WEEK 26	TIME	NOTES
MON		
TUE		
WED		
THU		
FRI		
SAT		
SUN		

WEEK 27	TIME	NOTES
MON		
TUE		
WED		
THU		
FRI		
SAT		
SUN		

WEEK 28	TIME	NOTES
MON		
TUE		
WED		
THU		
FRI		
SAT		
SUN		

WEEK 29	TIME	NOTES
MON		
TUE		
WED		
THU		
FRI		
SAT		
SUN		

WEEK 30	TIME	NOTES
MON		
TUE		
WED		
THU		
FRI		
SAT		
SUN		

WEEK 31	TIME	NOTES
MON		
TUE		
WED		
THU		
FRI		
SAT		
SUN		

WEEK 32	TIME	NOTES
MON		
TUE		
WED		
THU		
FRI		
SAT		
SUN		

WEEK 33	TIME	NOTES
MON		
TUE		
WED		
THU		
FRI		
SAT		
SUN		

Tracker

FETAL Movement

WEEK 34	TIME	NOTES
MON		
TUE		
WED		
THU		
FRI		
SAT		
SUN		

WEEK 35	TIME	NOTES
MON		
TUE		
WED		
THU		
FRI		
SAT		
SUN		

WEEK 36	TIME	NOTES
MON		
TUE		
WED		
THU		
FRI		
SAT		
SUN		

WEEK 37	TIME	NOTES
MON		
TUE		
WED		
THU		
FRI		
SAT		
SUN		

WEEK 38	TIME	NOTES
MON		
TUE		
WED		
THU		
FRI		
SAT		
SUN		

WEEK 39	TIME	NOTES
MON		
TUE		
WED		
THU		
FRI		
SAT		
SUN		

WEEK 40	TIME	NOTES
MON		
TUE		
WED		
THU		
FRI		
SAT		
SUN		

NOTES		

Week 4

PREGNANCY *Journal*

Your baby is the size of a poppy seed!

TOTAL
WEIGHT GAIN

BELLY
MEASUREMENT

BABY BUMP PHOTO

WEEKLY REFLECTIONS

SYMPTOMS & CRAVINGS

WHAT I WANT TO REMEMBER MOST

I'M MOST EXCITED ABOUT

I'M MOST NERVOUS ABOUT

Dear Baby,

Dear Baby

PREGNANCY *Journal*

TODAY'S DATE

WEEKS PREGNANT

HOW I'M FEELING TODAY

What I want you to know

Week 5

PREGNANCY Journal

Your baby is the size of a peppercorn!

TOTAL WEIGHT GAIN

BELLY MEASUREMENT

BABY BUMP PHOTO

WEEKLY REFLECTIONS

SYMPTOMS & CRAVINGS

WHAT I WANT TO REMEMBER MOST

I'M MOST EXCITED ABOUT

I'M MOST NERVOUS ABOUT

Dear Baby,

Dear Baby

PREGNANCY *Journal*

TODAY'S DATE

WEEKS PREGNANT

HOW I'M FEELING TODAY

What I want you to know

Week 6

PREGNANCY *Journal*

Your baby is the size of a sweet pea!

TOTAL WEIGHT GAIN

BELLY MEASUREMENT

BABY BUMP PHOTO

WEEKLY REFLECTIONS

SYMPTOMS & CRAVINGS

WHAT I WANT TO REMEMBER MOST

I'M MOST EXCITED ABOUT

I'M MOST NERVOUS ABOUT

Dear Baby,

Dear Baby

PREGNANCY *Journal*

TODAY'S
DATE

WEEKS
PREGNANT

HOW I'M
FEELING TODAY

What I want you to know

PREGNANCY *Journal*

Your baby is the size of a blueberry!

TOTAL WEIGHT GAIN	BELLY MEASUREMENT

WEEKLY REFLECTIONS

BABY BUMP PHOTO

SYMPTOMS & CRAVINGS

WHAT I WANT TO REMEMBER MOST

Dear Baby,

I'M MOST EXCITED ABOUT

I'M MOST NERVOUS ABOUT

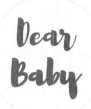

PREGNANCY *Journal*

TODAY'S
DATE

WEEKS
PREGNANT

HOW I'M
FEELING TODAY

What I want you to know

Week 8

PREGNANCY *Journal*

Your baby is the size of a raspberry!

TOTAL WEIGHT GAIN

BELLY MEASUREMENT

BABY BUMP PHOTO

WEEKLY REFLECTIONS

SYMPTOMS & CRAVINGS

WHAT I WANT TO REMEMBER MOST

Dear Baby,

I'M MOST EXCITED ABOUT

I'M MOST NERVOUS ABOUT

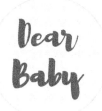

PREGNANCY *Journal*

TODAY'S
DATE

WEEKS
PREGNANT

HOW I'M
FEELING TODAY

What I want you to know

Week 9

PREGNANCY *Journal*

Your baby is the size of a grape!

TOTAL
WEIGHT GAIN

BELLY
MEASUREMENT

BABY BUMP PHOTO

WEEKLY REFLECTIONS

SYMPTOMS & CRAVINGS

WHAT I WANT TO REMEMBER MOST

Dear Baby,

I'M MOST EXCITED ABOUT

I'M MOST NERVOUS ABOUT

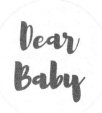

PREGNANCY *Journal*

TODAY'S
DATE

WEEKS
PREGNANT

HOW I'M
FEELING TODAY

What I want you to know

Week 10

PREGNANCY *Journal*

Your baby is the size of a prune!

TOTAL WEIGHT GAIN

BELLY MEASUREMENT

BABY BUMP PHOTO

WEEKLY REFLECTIONS

SYMPTOMS & CRAVINGS

WHAT I WANT TO REMEMBER MOST

Dear Baby,

I'M MOST EXCITED ABOUT

I'M MOST NERVOUS ABOUT

Dear Baby

PREGNANCY *Journal*

TODAY'S DATE

WEEKS PREGNANT

HOW I'M FEELING TODAY

What I want you to know

Week 11

PREGNANCY *Journal*

Your baby is the size of a lime!

TOTAL
WEIGHT GAIN

BELLY
MEASUREMENT

BABY BUMP PHOTO

WEEKLY REFLECTIONS

SYMPTOMS & CRAVINGS

WHAT I WANT TO REMEMBER MOST

Dear Baby,

I'M MOST EXCITED ABOUT

I'M MOST NERVOUS ABOUT

Dear Baby

PREGNANCY Journal

TODAY'S
DATE

WEEKS
PREGNANT

HOW I'M
FEELING TODAY

What I want you to know

Week 12

PREGNANCY *Journal*

Your baby is the size of a plum!

TOTAL WEIGHT GAIN

BELLY MEASUREMENT

BABY BUMP PHOTO

WEEKLY REFLECTIONS

SYMPTOMS & CRAVINGS

WHAT I WANT TO REMEMBER MOST

Dear Baby,

I'M MOST EXCITED ABOUT

I'M MOST NERVOUS ABOUT

12 WEEKS

ULTRASOUND Scan

ULTRASOUND PHOTO

ULTRASOUND RESULTS

BABY'S LENGTH:

BABY'S WEIGHT:

BPD:

DUE DATE:

Notes

Dear Baby

PREGNANCY *Journal*

TODAY'S DATE

WEEKS PREGNANT

HOW I'M FEELING TODAY

What I want you to know

Week 13

PREGNANCY *Journal*

Your baby is the size of a peach!

TOTAL WEIGHT GAIN	BELLY MEASUREMENT

WEEKLY REFLECTIONS

SYMPTOMS & CRAVINGS

BABY BUMP PHOTO

WHAT I WANT TO REMEMBER MOST

I'M MOST EXCITED ABOUT

I'M MOST NERVOUS ABOUT

Dear Baby,

Dear Baby

PREGNANCY Journal

TODAY'S
DATE

WEEKS
PREGNANT

HOW I'M
FEELING TODAY

What I want you to know

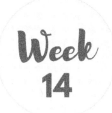

Week 14

PREGNANCY *Journal*

Your baby is the size of a lemon!

TOTAL
WEIGHT GAIN

BELLY
MEASUREMENT

BABY BUMP PHOTO

WEEKLY REFLECTIONS

SYMPTOMS & CRAVINGS

WHAT I WANT TO REMEMBER MOST

I'M MOST EXCITED ABOUT

I'M MOST NERVOUS ABOUT

Dear Baby,

Dear Baby

PREGNANCY *Journal*

TODAY'S DATE

WEEKS PREGNANT

HOW I'M FEELING TODAY

What I want you to know

Week 15

PREGNANCY *Journal*

Your baby is the size of an apple!

TOTAL
WEIGHT GAIN

BELLY
MEASUREMENT

BABY BUMP PHOTO

WEEKLY REFLECTIONS

SYMPTOMS & CRAVINGS

WHAT I WANT TO REMEMBER MOST

Dear Baby,

I'M MOST EXCITED ABOUT

I'M MOST NERVOUS ABOUT

Dear Baby

PREGNANCY *Journal*

TODAY'S
DATE

WEEKS
PREGNANT

HOW I'M
FEELING TODAY

What I want you to know

Week 16

PREGNANCY *Journal*

Your baby is the size of an avocado!

TOTAL WEIGHT GAIN

BELLY MEASUREMENT

BABY BUMP PHOTO

WEEKLY REFLECTIONS

SYMPTOMS & CRAVINGS

WHAT I WANT TO REMEMBER MOST

I'M MOST EXCITED ABOUT

I'M MOST NERVOUS ABOUT

Dear Baby,

Dear Baby

PREGNANCY *Journal*

TODAY'S
DATE

WEEKS
PREGNANT

HOW I'M
FEELING TODAY

What I want you to know

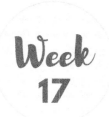

Week 17

PREGNANCY *Journal*

Your baby is the size of a pear!

TOTAL
WEIGHT GAIN

BELLY
MEASUREMENT

BABY BUMP PHOTO

WEEKLY REFLECTIONS

SYMPTOMS & CRAVINGS

WHAT I WANT TO REMEMBER MOST

I'M MOST EXCITED ABOUT

I'M MOST NERVOUS ABOUT

Dear Baby,

Dear Baby

PREGNANCY *Journal*

TODAY'S DATE

WEEKS PREGNANT

HOW I'M FEELING TODAY

What I want you to know

Week 18

PREGNANCY *Journal*

Your baby is the size of a sweet potato!

TOTAL
WEIGHT GAIN

BELLY
MEASUREMENT

BABY BUMP PHOTO

WEEKLY REFLECTIONS

SYMPTOMS & CRAVINGS

WHAT I WANT TO REMEMBER MOST

Dear Baby,

I'M MOST EXCITED ABOUT

I'M MOST NERVOUS ABOUT

Dear Baby

PREGNANCY *Journal*

TODAY'S DATE

WEEKS PREGNANT

HOW I'M FEELING TODAY

What I want you to know

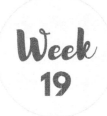

Week 19

PREGNANCY *Journal*

Your baby is the size of a mango!

TOTAL WEIGHT GAIN

BELLY MEASUREMENT

BABY BUMP PHOTO

WEEKLY REFLECTIONS

SYMPTOMS & CRAVINGS

WHAT I WANT TO REMEMBER MOST

I'M MOST EXCITED ABOUT

I'M MOST NERVOUS ABOUT

Dear Baby,

Dear Baby

PREGNANCY *Journal*

TODAY'S
DATE

WEEKS
PREGNANT

HOW I'M
FEELING TODAY

What I want you to know

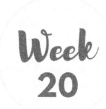

Week 20

PREGNANCY *Journal*

Your baby is the size of a banana!

TOTAL
WEIGHT GAIN

BELLY
MEASUREMENT

BABY BUMP PHOTO

WEEKLY REFLECTIONS

SYMPTOMS & CRAVINGS

WHAT I WANT TO REMEMBER MOST

I'M MOST EXCITED ABOUT

I'M MOST NERVOUS ABOUT

Dear Baby,

20 WEEKS

ULTRASOUND Scan

ULTRASOUND PHOTO

ULTRASOUND RESULTS

BABY'S LENGTH:

BABY'S WEIGHT:

BPD:

DUE DATE:

Notes

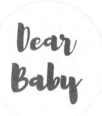

PREGNANCY *Journal*

TODAY'S
DATE

WEEKS
PREGNANT

HOW I'M
FEELING TODAY

What I want you to know

Week 21

PREGNANCY *Journal*

Your baby is the size of a carrot!

TOTAL WEIGHT GAIN

BELLY MEASUREMENT

BABY BUMP PHOTO

WEEKLY REFLECTIONS

SYMPTOMS & CRAVINGS

WHAT I WANT TO REMEMBER MOST

I'M MOST EXCITED ABOUT

I'M MOST NERVOUS ABOUT

Dear Baby,

Dear Baby

PREGNANCY *Journal*

**TODAY'S
DATE**

**WEEKS
PREGNANT**

**HOW I'M
FEELING TODAY**

What I want you to know

Week 22

PREGNANCY *Journal*

Your baby is the size of a papaya!

TOTAL WEIGHT GAIN

BELLY MEASUREMENT

BABY BUMP PHOTO

WEEKLY REFLECTIONS

SYMPTOMS & CRAVINGS

WHAT I WANT TO REMEMBER MOST

Dear Baby,

I'M MOST EXCITED ABOUT

I'M MOST NERVOUS ABOUT

Dear Baby

PREGNANCY *Journal*

TODAY'S
DATE

WEEKS
PREGNANT

HOW I'M
FEELING TODAY

What I want you to know

PREGNANCY *Journal*

Your baby is the size of a grapefruit!

TOTAL
WEIGHT GAIN

BELLY
MEASUREMENT

BABY BUMP PHOTO

WEEKLY REFLECTIONS

SYMPTOMS & CRAVINGS

WHAT I WANT TO REMEMBER MOST

Dear Baby,

I'M MOST EXCITED ABOUT

I'M MOST NERVOUS ABOUT

Dear Baby

PREGNANCY Journal

TODAY'S DATE

WEEKS PREGNANT

HOW I'M FEELING TODAY

What I want you to know

Week 24

PREGNANCY *Journal*

Your baby is the size of a cantaloupe!

TOTAL WEIGHT GAIN

BELLY MEASUREMENT

BABY BUMP PHOTO

WEEKLY REFLECTIONS

SYMPTOMS & CRAVINGS

WHAT I WANT TO REMEMBER MOST

I'M MOST EXCITED ABOUT

I'M MOST NERVOUS ABOUT

Dear Baby,

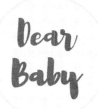

Dear Baby

PREGNANCY *Journal*

TODAY'S
DATE

WEEKS
PREGNANT

HOW I'M
FEELING TODAY

What I want you to know

PREGNANCY *Journal*

Your baby is the size of a cauliflower!

TOTAL
WEIGHT GAIN

BELLY
MEASUREMENT

BABY BUMP PHOTO

WEEKLY REFLECTIONS

SYMPTOMS & CRAVINGS

WHAT I WANT TO REMEMBER MOST

Dear Baby,

I'M MOST EXCITED ABOUT

I'M MOST NERVOUS ABOUT

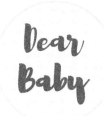

PREGNANCY *Journal*

TODAY'S
DATE

WEEKS
PREGNANT

HOW I'M
FEELING TODAY

What I want you to know

Week 26

PREGNANCY *Journal*

Your baby is the size of a head of lettuce!

TOTAL
WEIGHT GAIN

BELLY
MEASUREMENT

BABY BUMP PHOTO

WEEKLY REFLECTIONS

SYMPTOMS & CRAVINGS

WHAT I WANT TO REMEMBER MOST

Dear Baby,

I'M MOST EXCITED ABOUT

I'M MOST NERVOUS ABOUT

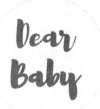

PREGNANCY *Journal*

TODAY'S DATE	WEEKS PREGNANT	HOW I'M FEELING TODAY

What I want you to know

Week 27

PREGNANCY *Journal*

Your baby is the size of a rutabaga!

TOTAL WEIGHT GAIN	BELLY MEASUREMENT

WEEKLY REFLECTIONS

SYMPTOMS & CRAVINGS

WHAT I WANT TO REMEMBER MOST

I'M MOST EXCITED ABOUT

I'M MOST NERVOUS ABOUT

BABY BUMP PHOTO

Dear Baby,

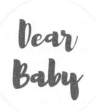

PREGNANCY *Journal*

TODAY'S DATE

WEEKS PREGNANT

HOW I'M FEELING TODAY

What I want you to know

Week 28

PREGNANCY *Journal*

Your baby is the size of an eggplant!

TOTAL
WEIGHT GAIN

BELLY
MEASUREMENT

BABY BUMP PHOTO

WEEKLY REFLECTIONS

SYMPTOMS & CRAVINGS

WHAT I WANT TO REMEMBER MOST

Dear Baby,

I'M MOST EXCITED ABOUT

I'M MOST NERVOUS ABOUT

Dear Baby

PREGNANCY *Journal*

♥ ♥ ♥ ♥ ♥ ♥ ♥ ♥ ♥ ♥ ♥ ♥ ♥ ♥ ♥ ♥ ♥ ♥

TODAY'S
DATE

WEEKS
PREGNANT

HOW I'M
FEELING TODAY

What I want you to know

Week 29

PREGNANCY *Journal*

Your baby is the size of an acorn squash!

TOTAL WEIGHT GAIN

BELLY MEASUREMENT

BABY BUMP PHOTO

WEEKLY REFLECTIONS

SYMPTOMS & CRAVINGS

WHAT I WANT TO REMEMBER MOST

I'M MOST EXCITED ABOUT

I'M MOST NERVOUS ABOUT

Dear Baby,

Dear Baby

PREGNANCY *Journal*

♥ ♥ ♥ ♥ ♥ ♥ ♥ ♥ ♥ ♥ ♥ ♥ ♥ ♥ ♥ ♥ ♥ ♥ ♥ ♥

TODAY'S DATE

WEEKS PREGNANT

HOW I'M FEELING TODAY

What I want you to know

Week 30

PREGNANCY *Journal*

Your baby is the size of a cucumber!

TOTAL WEIGHT GAIN	BELLY MEASUREMENT

BABY BUMP PHOTO

WEEKLY REFLECTIONS

SYMPTOMS & CRAVINGS

WHAT I WANT TO REMEMBER MOST

I'M MOST EXCITED ABOUT

I'M MOST NERVOUS ABOUT

Dear Baby,

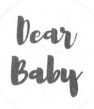

PREGNANCY *Journal*

TODAY'S
DATE

WEEKS
PREGNANT

HOW I'M
FEELING TODAY

What I want you to know

Week 31

PREGNANCY *Journal*

Your baby is the size of a pineapple!

TOTAL WEIGHT GAIN

BELLY MEASUREMENT

BABY BUMP PHOTO

WEEKLY REFLECTIONS

SYMPTOMS & CRAVINGS

WHAT I WANT TO REMEMBER MOST

I'M MOST EXCITED ABOUT

I'M MOST NERVOUS ABOUT

Dear Baby,

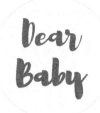

PREGNANCY *Journal*

TODAY'S DATE

WEEKS PREGNANT

HOW I'M FEELING TODAY

What I want you to know

Week 32

PREGNANCY *Journal*

Your baby is the size of a squash!

TOTAL WEIGHT GAIN

BELLY MEASUREMENT

BABY BUMP PHOTO

WEEKLY REFLECTIONS

SYMPTOMS & CRAVINGS

WHAT I WANT TO REMEMBER MOST

I'M MOST EXCITED ABOUT

I'M MOST NERVOUS ABOUT

Dear Baby,

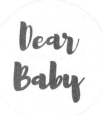

PREGNANCY *Journal*

TODAY'S DATE	WEEKS PREGNANT	HOW I'M FEELING TODAY

What I want you to know

Week 33

PREGNANCY Journal

Your baby is the size of a durian!

TOTAL WEIGHT GAIN

BELLY MEASUREMENT

BABY BUMP PHOTO

WEEKLY REFLECTIONS

SYMPTOMS & CRAVINGS

WHAT I WANT TO REMEMBER MOST

Dear Baby,

I'M MOST EXCITED ABOUT

I'M MOST NERVOUS ABOUT

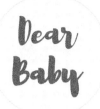

PREGNANCY *Journal*

TODAY'S
DATE

WEEKS
PREGNANT

HOW I'M
FEELING TODAY

What I want you to know

Week 34

PREGNANCY *Journal*

Your baby is the size of a butternut squash!

TOTAL WEIGHT GAIN

BELLY MEASUREMENT

BABY BUMP PHOTO

WEEKLY REFLECTIONS

SYMPTOMS & CRAVINGS

WHAT I WANT TO REMEMBER MOST

I'M MOST EXCITED ABOUT

I'M MOST NERVOUS ABOUT

Dear Baby,

Dear Baby

PREGNANCY Journal

TODAY'S
DATE

WEEKS
PREGNANT

HOW I'M
FEELING TODAY

What I want you to know

PREGNANCY *Journal*

Your baby is the size of a coconut!

TOTAL
WEIGHT GAIN

BELLY
MEASUREMENT

BABY BUMP PHOTO

WEEKLY REFLECTIONS

SYMPTOMS & CRAVINGS

WHAT I WANT TO REMEMBER MOST

Dear Baby,

I'M MOST EXCITED ABOUT

I'M MOST NERVOUS ABOUT

Dear Baby

PREGNANCY *Journal*

TODAY'S
DATE

WEEKS
PREGNANT

HOW I'M
FEELING TODAY

What I want you to know

Week 36

PREGNANCY *Journal*

Your baby is the size of a honeydew melon!

TOTAL
WEIGHT GAIN

BELLY
MEASUREMENT

BABY BUMP PHOTO

WEEKLY REFLECTIONS

SYMPTOMS & CRAVINGS

WHAT I WANT TO REMEMBER MOST

Dear Baby,

I'M MOST EXCITED ABOUT

I'M MOST NERVOUS ABOUT

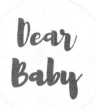

PREGNANCY *Journal*

TODAY'S DATE

WEEKS PREGNANT

HOW I'M FEELING TODAY

What I want you to know

Week 37

PREGNANCY *Journal*

Your baby is the size of a Winter Melon!

TOTAL WEIGHT GAIN

BELLY MEASUREMENT

BABY BUMP PHOTO

WEEKLY REFLECTIONS

SYMPTOMS & CRAVINGS

WHAT I WANT TO REMEMBER MOST

Dear Baby,

I'M MOST EXCITED ABOUT

I'M MOST NERVOUS ABOUT

Dear Baby

PREGNANCY Journal

TODAY'S
DATE

WEEKS
PREGNANT

HOW I'M
FEELING TODAY

What I want you to know

Week 38

PREGNANCY *Journal*

Your baby is the size of a pumpkin!

TOTAL WEIGHT GAIN	BELLY MEASUREMENT

BABY BUMP PHOTO

WEEKLY REFLECTIONS

SYMPTOMS & CRAVINGS

WHAT I WANT TO REMEMBER MOST

Dear Baby,

I'M MOST EXCITED ABOUT

I'M MOST NERVOUS ABOUT

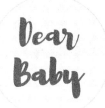

PREGNANCY *Journal*

TODAY'S
DATE

WEEKS
PREGNANT

HOW I'M
FEELING TODAY

What I want you to know

Week 39

PREGNANCY *Journal*

Your baby is the size of a watermelon!

TOTAL WEIGHT GAIN

BELLY MEASUREMENT

BABY BUMP PHOTO

WEEKLY REFLECTIONS

SYMPTOMS & CRAVINGS

WHAT I WANT TO REMEMBER MOST

I'M MOST EXCITED ABOUT

I'M MOST NERVOUS ABOUT

Dear Baby,

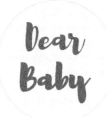

PREGNANCY *Journal*

TODAY'S
DATE

WEEKS
PREGNANT

HOW I'M
FEELING TODAY

What I want you to know

Week 40

PREGNANCY Journal

Your baby is the size of a jack fruit!

TOTAL WEIGHT GAIN	BELLY MEASUREMENT

WEEKLY REFLECTIONS

SYMPTOMS & CRAVINGS

WHAT I WANT TO REMEMBER MOST

I'M MOST EXCITED ABOUT

I'M MOST NERVOUS ABOUT

BABY BUMP PHOTO

Dear Baby,

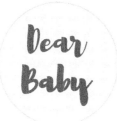

PREGNANCY *Journal*

TODAY'S DATE

WEEKS PREGNANT

HOW I'M FEELING TODAY

What I want you to know

Made in the USA
Middletown, DE
10 November 2022

14534466R00057